CONQUERING COLORECTAL CANCER

Empowering Strategies, Expert Advice, and Awareness for Overcoming Colon Cancer and Reclaiming Your Life

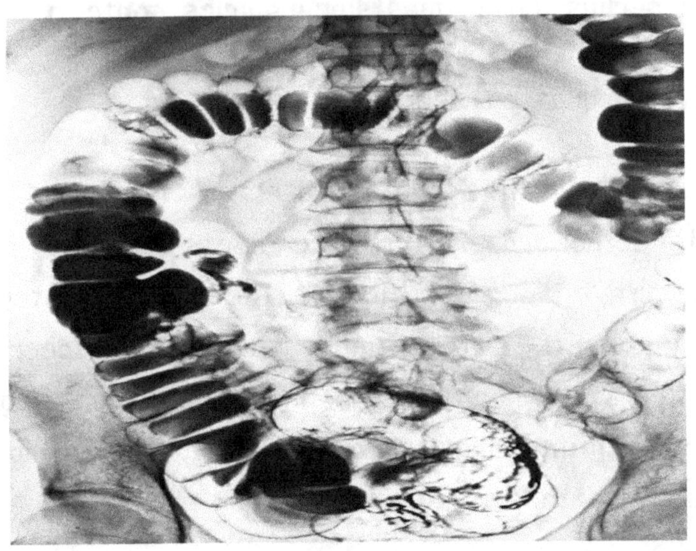

Dr. Marquette Gw

Contents

- Flexible Sigmoidoscopy:

- Colonoscopy:

- CT Colonography:

Diagnostic tests

- Colonoscopy:

- Biopsy:

- Blood Tests:

- Imaging Tests:

Staging: What It Means

- T (Tumor)

- N (Nodes)

- M (Metastasis)

Therapeutic Options for Colorectal Cancer

Surgery

The Functions of Support Groups and Counseling

Lifestyle and Prevention: A Guide to Lowering Colorectal Cancer Risk

Diet & Nutrition

- Reduce Consumption of Red and Processed Meats:

- Incorporate Dairy:

Exertion and Physical Activity

- Stay Active:

- Muscle Strength:

Preventive measures and screenings

- Regular Screenings

- Screening Types

RECOMMENDED DIET RECIPES

Survivorship and Beyond: Navigating Life Following Colorectal Cancer Treatment

Life Following Treatment

- Re-establish Routines:

- Monitor Health:

- Embrace Changes:

Manage Long-Term Side Effects

- Fatigue:

- Neuropathy:

- Digestive Changes:

Importance of Follow-Up Care

- Regular Screenings:

- Monitoring for Recurrence

- Personal Health Records:

Embrace the Future with Hope and Courage

Awareness and Early Detection:

Understanding the Disease:

Diagnosis and Staging:

Treatment Options:

Navigating the Healthcare System:

The Patient's Journey:

Lifestyle and Prevention:

Survivorship and Beyond:

INTRODUCTION

Colorectal cancer is the world's third most frequent cancer and the second greatest cause of cancer-related deaths. Despite its prevalence, the fight against this disease is not hopeless. The strength of awareness and early detection is the key to overcoming colorectal cancer.

The Value of Awareness and Early Detection

Awareness is our first line of defense. It provides individuals with the knowledge they need to identify the risk factors and symptoms linked with colorectal cancer. Screenings are crucial, especially in the United States, where over 150,000 new diagnoses occur annually. Early detection through regular screenings can significantly raise the likelihood of successful treatment and survival. The Blue March highlights the importance of early detection and encourages individuals to take proactive actions in their health journey.

Screening is a source of hope, showing the route to early intervention. Early detection of colorectal cancer leads to more successful and less intrusive therapy. The Westchester County Department of Health and other health groups promote frequent screenings as a life-saving measure.

An Overview of Colorectal Cancer

Colorectal cancer begins its insidious trip in the colon or rectum, usually without warning. In the early stages, symptoms may be absent, making tests even more important. As the condition advances, symptoms may include changes in bowel habits, blood in the stool, and unexplained weight loss.

Colorectal cancer develops in a complex manner, frequently beginning with benign polyps that might progress to malignant tumors over time. Various factors, including age, family history, lifestyle, and genetics, can dramatically impact risk. The World Health

Organization recommends healthy habits and regular tests as major preventative strategies.

As we progress through this book, we will look deeper into every facet of colorectal cancer, from diagnosis to survivorship. We will look at empowering tactics, professional guidance, and real-life examples that will not only educate but also inspire. Together, we will face challenges and enjoy victories on the way to reclaiming life from colorectal cancer.

This introduction sets the tone for a book that seeks to educate, motivate, and empower readers to take control of their health and overcome colorectal cancer.

Understanding Colorectal Cancer

Colorectal cancer is a common, possibly fatal disease that affects the colon and rectum. Uncontrolled cell proliferation in the colon or rectum can cause tumors and spread throughout the body. Understanding the condition is critical for prevention, early discovery, and successful treatment.

What is colorectal cancer?

Colorectal cancer begins with benign polyps in the large intestine or rectum and can progress to malignancy over time. It is commonly known as colon cancer when it affects the colon and rectal cancer when it affects the rectum. The condition can impair the digestive system's waste processing, resulting in serious health complications.

Causes and risk factors

Although the precise origin of colorectal cancer remains unknown, numerous risk factors have been identified:

- Mutations in the DNA of colon or rectal cells can cause aberrant cell growth.
- Lifestyle variables include high-fat, low-fiber diet, lack of physical activity, obesity, smoking, and excessive alcohol intake can all raise the risk.

- The majority of occurrences occur in those over 50 years old.
- Family history and genetic disorders, such as Lynch syndrome and familial adenomatous polyposis (FAP), play a role.

Signs and Symptoms To Watch For

Early-stage colorectal cancer may not cause any symptoms. However, as the condition advances, a number of indications and symptoms may appear:

- Bowel habits changes, such diarrhea or constipation.
- Blood in the feces might cause it to appear dark brown or black.

- Symptoms include abdominal discomfort, cramps, gas, or pain.

- Feeling that the intestines does not fully empty with a bowel movement.

- unexplained weight loss, weakness, and exhaustion.

If any of these symptoms continue, you should see a doctor right away because early discovery can dramatically enhance treatment outcomes. Regular checkups and a healthy lifestyle are critical components in the fight against colorectal cancer. Understanding the condition, its origins, and symptoms allows people to take proactive efforts to lower their risk and seek medical assistance as needed.

Diagnosis and staging of colorectal cancer

The path to overcoming colorectal cancer begins with a precise diagnosis and comprehension of the disease's stage. This information is critical for determining the best effective treatment approach.

Screening Methods

Screening for colorectal cancer is a proactive measure that detects the disease before symptoms develop. Several approaches are recommended, such as:

- **Stool Tests:** Options include the guaiac-based fecal occult blood test (gFOBT), fecal immunochemical test (FIT), and multitargeted stool DNA test (FIT-DNA).

- **Flexible Sigmoidoscopy:** A flexible, lighted tube inspects the rectum and lower third of the colon every 5 years, or every 10 years with a FIT every year.

- **Colonoscopy:** Examines the entire colon and rectum every 10 years for people at average risk.

- **CT Colonography:** Every 5 years, often known as virtual colonoscopy.

Diagnostic tests

If screening findings indicate colorectal cancer, or if symptoms exist, more diagnostic tests are performed such as:

- Colonoscopy: Enables visual examination and biopsy of polyps.

- Biopsy: Tissue samples are collected for histological evaluation.

- Blood Tests: Comprehensive blood count (CBC) and liver function tests to evaluate overall health and tumor indicators including carcinoembryonic antigen (CEA).

- Imaging Tests: CT scans, MRIs, and ultrasounds can visualize the tumor and detect spread.

Staging: What It Means

The TNM system determines staging, which represents the amount of cancer in the body.

- T (Tumor) indicates the size and extent of the main tumor.
- N (Nodes) indicates the absence or presence of regional lymph node involvement.
- M (Metastasis) indicates whether the cancer has migrated to other places of the body.

Cancer stages range from 0 (no growth beyond the mucosa) to IV (cancer has spread to distant organs). Each stage directs treatment and affects prognosis.

Understanding the diagnosis and staging of colorectal cancer is an important step in the fight against the illness. Patients and healthcare providers can collaborate to establish a specific treatment strategy that gives them the best chance of success.

Therapeutic Options for Colorectal Cancer

Colorectal cancer treatment consists of a variety of treatments that can be employed alone or in combination, depending on the cancer's stage and characteristics. Here's an outline of the main therapy choices.

Surgery

Surgery is frequently the first line treatment for colorectal cancer. It can range from minimally invasive approaches, such eliminating polyps during a colonoscopy, to more complex surgeries, such as partial or total colectomy.

Lymph nodes around a tumor are typically removed for examination.

Chemotherapy

Chemotherapy is a drug-based treatment that is usually used following surgery to remove any leftover cancer cells. It can decrease tumors prior to surgery, making them easier to remove. Common medicines are 5-fluorouracil, capecitabine, and oxaliplatin.

Radiation therapy

Radiation therapy employs high-energy beams to attack cancer cells. It is more usually used to treat rectal cancer than colon cancer.

Radiation can be delivered externally or internally, and it is frequently combined with chemotherapy to improve its effectiveness.

Targeted therapy

Targeted treatment medications function by concentrating on certain genetic targets found in cancer cells. Drugs such as bevacizumab and cetuximab target proteins that aid cancer cell growth and spread. Combining these treatments with chemotherapy is common for advanced malignancies.

Immunotherapy

Immunotherapy strengthens the body's immune system to combat cancer. Colorectal tumors with certain genetic characteristics, such as high microsatellite instability or mismatch repair deficiency, can benefit from drugs like pembrolizumab and nivolumab.

Alternative treatments

Alternative therapies, while not a replacement for traditional treatment, can assist control symptoms and improve quality of life. These may include acupuncture, massage, herbal supplements, and dietary adjustments. It's important to examine these possibilities with a healthcare physician to ensure they don't interfere with normal treatments.

Each treatment strategy has possible benefits and hazards, and the ideal technique is determined by specific patient characteristics. You should review all available treatment choices with their healthcare team to identify the best plan for their unique condition.

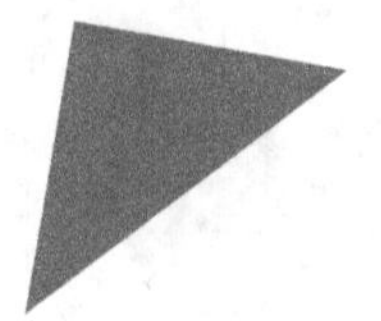

4

Navigating the Healthcare System

Navigating the healthcare system can be difficult, especially when faced with a colorectal cancer diagnosis. Here is a handbook to aid you along this journey:

Finding the Right Medical Team

Your medical team is your health partner, so choosing the proper professionals is critical. A multidisciplinary team often consists of medical oncologists, surgeons, radiation oncologists, and nurse specialists. Each has a particular role in your treatment and recovery. To find the appropriate team:

- Look for hospitals or clinics that offer comprehensive cancer care programs.
- Look for professionals who have experience treating colorectal cancer.
- Consider the medical team's communication style and availability.

Understanding Insurance and Costs

Cancer treatment can be costly, therefore it's important to understand your insurance coverage:

- Review your insurance policy to determine which therapies and medications are covered.
- Inquire with your healthcare practitioner about the expenses involved with different treatment options.
- Look into financial aid programs to help meet care costs.

Seeking Second Opinions

Obtaining a second opinion can provide reassurance or other treatment alternatives.

Patients have the right to seek a second opinion, and most doctors support this decision. A second opinion can confirm your diagnosis, provide additional information, or recommend alternative treatment options. Request a referral from your doctor or contact cancer centers that provide second opinions.

Navigating the healthcare system involves patience and tenacity, but being knowledgeable and proactive can help make the process go more smoothly and ensure that you get the best care available for your illness.

The Patient's Journey: Triumphs and Trials of Conquering Colorectal Cancer

The journey through colorectal cancer is a personal story of perseverance, demonstrating the human spirit's ability to overcome hardship. This chapter goes into patients' diverse experiences, the emotional journey of the diagnosis, and the critical function of support systems.

True-Life Stories of Diagnosis and Treatment

The tapestry of real-life stories provides a realistic picture of the colorectal cancer journey. From the initial shock of diagnosis to the grueling path of therapy, each story is distinct. Anatole Karpovs, a pediatrician with a medical education, struggled to accept his symptoms. Raquel's experience with dismissive healthcare personnel prior to her stage 4 diagnosis highlights the importance of advocating for and receiving appropriate care.

The Emotional Impact Of Cancer

A colon cancer diagnosis can cause an emotional cascade, eliciting feelings of fear, grief, and uncertainty. Patients' emotional well-being is equally important to their physical health. Many cancer survivors face long-term psychological issues, such as despair and anxiety, according to research. Recognizing these emotional responses is the first step toward recovery.

The Functions of Support Groups and Counseling

Support groups and counseling are the foundation of emotional rehabilitation, providing a safe space for expression and understanding. Patients can share their experiences and coping skills, creating a sense of collective strength. Counseling helps people negotiate their emotions and cope with cancer-related changes. Together, these support structures promote a sense of belonging, hope, and resilience.

Finally, the patient's experience through colorectal cancer is not unique. It is a shared journey, paved with the stories of fellow travelers, the empathy of support groups, and the advice of counselors. It is a courageous journey, one that continues to inspire and motivate people who embark on it.

Lifestyle and Prevention: A Guide to Lowering Colorectal Cancer Risk

The cliché "prevention is better than cure" rings especially true with colorectal cancer. Lifestyle changes can significantly reduce the likelihood of having this disease. Here's a complete look at food, exercise, and preventative strategies to help you avoid colorectal cancer.

Diet & Nutrition

A well-balanced diet is essential for preventing colorectal cancer. The dietary suggestions below are based on study findings:

Consuming whole grains, nuts, seeds, legumes, and a range of fruits and vegetables can greatly increase fiber intake, which is associated with a decreased risk of colorectal cancer.

- **Reduce Consumption of Red and Processed Meats:** Research indicates that limiting red meats like beef, hog, or lamb, as well as processed meats like hot dogs and luncheon meats, can lower the risk of colorectal cancer.
- **Incorporate Dairy:** Consuming enough dairy may help prevent colorectal cancer.
- Maintain colon health by being hydrated, especially with plenty of water.

Exertion and Physical Activity

Regular physical exercise is not only beneficial to overall health, but it is also an effective preventive measure against colorectal cancer.

- **Stay Active:** It is recommended that you engage in 30-60 minutes of moderate to strenuous physical activity every day. This can include any sort of activity that boosts heart rate, such as walking, cycling, and swimming.

- **Muscle Strength:** Exercise boosts muscle strength, which can be advantageous during and after cancer treatment.

Preventive measures and screenings

Early identification through screening is one of the most effective ways for preventing colorectal cancer.

- **Regular Screenings:** The U.S. Preventive Services Task Force recommends colorectal cancer screening for persons aged 45 to 75. Individuals between the ages of 76 and 85 should make their own screening decision.
- **Screening Types:** Several screening tests are available, including stool tests, flexible sigmoidoscopy, colonoscopy, and CT colonography (virtual colonoscopy).

Consult with your healthcare professional to determine which tests are appropriate for you.

RECOMMENDED DIET RECIPES

The following diet recipes are designed specifically for colorectal cancer patients, concentrating on nutritional requirements and ease of digestion. I'll also proffer the ingredients and methods for each recipe:

1. High-Protein Chicken and Vegetable Soup

Ingredients

- 2 chicken breasts, cubed.

- 1 cup diced carrots.

- One cup chopped celery

- 1/2 cup of diced onions.

- 4 cups low-sodium chicken broth.

- One teaspoon olive oil

- Add salt and pepper to taste.

- Fresh herbs (such as parsley) for garnish.

Preparation

1. Warm the olive oil in a big pot over medium heat.

2. Sauté the onions, carrots, and celery until they are transparent.

3. Cook the chicken cubes until no longer pink on the exterior.

4. Pour in the chicken broth and heat to a boil.

5. Reduce the heat to a simmer for 20 minutes, or until the veggies are soft.

6. Season with salt and pepper and serve with fresh herbs.

2. Quinoa with Roasted Vegetable Salad

Ingredients

- One cup quinoa

- 2 cups water.

- 1 cup chopped bell peppers.

- 1 cup halved cherry tomatoes.

- 1/2 cup of diced cucumbers.

- 1/4 cup of olive oil.

- Two tablespoons of lemon juice.

- Add salt and pepper to taste.

Preparation

1. Preheat your oven to 375°F (190°C).

2. Place the bell peppers and cherry tomatoes on a baking pan and drizzle with olive oil. Roast for 20 minutes.

3. Rinse the quinoa in cold water, then combine it with 2 cups of water in a saucepan. Bring to a boil, then cover and let simmer for 15 minutes.

4. Using a fork, fluff the cooked quinoa and allow it to cool.

5. In a large mixing dish, add the quinoa, roasted

veggies, and cucumbers.

6. Whisk together the olive oil and lemon juice, then pour over the salad and toss to incorporate. Season with salt and pepper to taste.

3. Ginger-Steamed Fish & Greens

Ingredients

- 4 fish fillets (cod or tilapia)

- One tablespoon grated ginger

- Two cups spinach or kale.

- One tablespoon of low-sodium soy sauce.

- One teaspoon of sesame oil.

Preparation

1. Place the fish fillets on a steamable plate.

2. Sprinkle the shredded ginger over the fish.

3. Prepare your steamer and set the plate of fish inside. Cover and steam for approximately 10 minutes, or until the fish flakes easily with a fork.

4. In the last 2 minutes of steaming, place the greens around the fish to lightly steam.

5. Season the fish and greens with soy sauce and sesame oil before serving.

4. Oatmeal with Berries and Nuts.

Ingredients

- One cup rolled oats.

- Two cups of water or milk.

- 1/2 cup mixed berries, fresh or frozen.

- $\frac{1}{4}$ cup chopped nuts (almonds or walnuts)

- Add honey or maple syrup to taste.

Preparation

1. In a saucepan, heat the water or milk to a boil.

2. Stir in the oats and decrease the heat to a simmer. Cook 5 minutes, stirring periodically.

3. Once the oats have cooked, remove them from the heat and set aside for 2 minutes.

4. Top the oats with berries, nuts, and a drizzle of honey or maple syrup.

5. Smoothie with Protein Powder

Ingredients

- 1 cup almond milk or another non-dairy milk.

- One banana.

- 1/2 cup of frozen mango pieces.

- One scoop of vanilla or unflavored protein powder.

- One tablespoon of almond butter.

Preparation

1. Combine all ingredients in a blender.

2. Blend on high until smooth and creamy.

3. Pour into a glass and drink immediately.

6. Creamy Greek Yogurt with Soft Fruits

Ingredients

- One cup plain Greek yogurt.

- 1/2 cup soft fruits, such as bananas or peaches.

- A sprinkle of honey or maple syrup.

Preparation

1. Add the Greek yogurt to a bowl.

2. Top with soft fruits.

3. Drizzle with honey or maple syrup, to taste.

7. Tender Turkey Meatballs

Ingredients

- 1 pound ground turkey.

-1/4 cup breadcrumbs

- 1 egg

- 1/4 cup grated parmesan cheese.

- Add salt and herbs to taste.

Preparation

1. Preheat your oven to 375°F (190°C).

2. In a mixing basin, combine all of the ingredients thoroughly.

3. Roll into tiny meatballs and lay them on a baking pan.

4. Bake for 20 to 25 minutes, or until thoroughly done.

8. Mashed Sweet Potatoes

Ingredients

- two huge sweet potatoes, peeled and cubed

- Two tablespoons butter.

- Add salt to taste.

Preparation

1. Boil sweet potatoes till soft.

2. Drain, then return to the pot.

3. Add the butter and mash until smooth.

4. Add salt to taste.

9. Baked Salmon with Lemon

Ingredients

-4 salmon fillets

- two lemons, cut

- Olive Oil

- Add salt and pepper to taste.

Preparation

1. Preheat your oven to 400°F (200°C).

2. Place the salmon on a baking sheet, then top

with lemon slices.

3. Drizzle with olive oil, then season with salt and pepper.

4. Bake for 12-15 minutes, or until the fish flakes easily.

10. Avocado and Egg Toast

Ingredients

- 2 pieces of white bread, toasted

- One ripe avocado.

- Two soft-boiled or poached eggs.

- Add salt and pepper to taste.

Preparation

1. Mash the avocado and spread it on bread.

2. Top with eggs.

3. Add salt and pepper to taste.

Individuals can dramatically lower their risk of colorectal cancer by eating a nutritious diet, exercising regularly, and getting frequent screenings. These lifestyle changes are within most people's reach and can make a significant difference in the fight against this disease.

Survivorship and Beyond: Navigating Life Following Colorectal Cancer Treatment

Surviving colorectal cancer is a huge accomplishment, but the road does not stop with the final treatment. The path to recovery can be long, and understanding how to navigate life after treatment is critical for sustaining health and well-being.

Life Following Treatment

After finishing treatment, many survivors must adjust to a new normal. Adjusting to changes in physical ability, energy levels, and daily routines can take some time. It is crucial to:

- **Re-establish Routines:** Gradually returning to pre-cancer activities can aid in restoring a sense of normalcy.

- **Monitor Health:** Regular check-ups are crucial to identify any difficulties early.

- **Embrace Changes:** Adapting to changes in your body and lifestyle can promote personal growth and fulfillment.

Manage Long-Term Side Effects

Colorectal cancer treatment might cause survivors to experience long-term adverse effects such as:

- **Fatigue:** This is a very common adverse effect. Managing energy levels through rest and moderate activity can be beneficial.

- **Neuropathy:** Chemotherapy can induce nerve damage, resulting in tingling or numbness, particularly in the hands and feet. Physical therapy and medicines can help relieve symptoms.

- **Digestive Changes**: Bowel changes are prevalent. Dietary changes and drugs can alleviate these symptoms.

Importance of Follow-Up Care

Follow-up care is essential for monitoring recovery and detecting any return of cancer early.

- **Regular Screenings**: Colonoscopies and other testing detect any new alterations in the colon or rectum.
- **Monitoring for Recurrence**: Keeping an eye out for symptoms and attending all follow-up appointments can detect

recurrences early when they are most treatable.

- **Personal Health Records:** Maintaining detailed health records will assist you and your healthcare team in making educated decisions about your car.

Survivorship is a demonstration of strength and resilience. With the correct methods and support, survivors can flourish following colorectal cancer therapy.

Conclusion

Embrace the Future with Hope and Courage

As we conclude our journey through "Conquering Colorectal Cancer," it's vital to reflect on the major concepts that have served as the foundation of this guide:

Awareness and Early Detection: It is impossible to overstate the importance of awareness and the possibility for saving lives.

Understanding the Disease: Knowing what colorectal cancer is, its causes, risk factors, and symptoms is critical for prevention and early treatment.

Diagnosis and Staging: Knowing the stage of cancer is critical for optimal treatment planning.

Treatment Options: A variety of treatments, including surgery and immunotherapy, give hope for recovery and disease management.

Navigating the Healthcare System: Understanding how to navigate the healthcare system, identify the correct medical team, and manage insurance and costs is a key to empowerment.

The Patient's Journey: Cancer has a profound emotional impact, and support groups and counseling are helpful.

Lifestyle and Prevention: Maintaining a healthy lifestyle and scheduling frequent screenings are effective prevention techniques.

Survivorship and Beyond: Life following treatment entails dealing with long-term adverse effects and comprehending the value of follow-up care.

As you're going on this journey, you must realize that you are not alone. Many people who have walked this path before you, as well as those who are now walking beside you, share your experience. Allow their stories to inspire you, knowledge to strengthen you, and courage to be the light that guides you forward.

Remember that every step forward brings us closer to a future in which colorectal cancer is not the end of the journey, but rather a part of a greater story of survival and optimism. Stand tall, for you are a shining example of resilience. Carry on with determination, for every day brings new opportunities. Above all, cling on to hope, since it is the anchor that will keep you on track toward reclaiming your life.

May this book serve as a compass, a source of information, and a tribute to your inner power. Forge ahead with courage, because your narrative is one of success and encouragement to everybody.

CHECK OUT THESE OTHER BOOKS

www.ingramcontent.com/pod-product-compliance
Lightning Source LLC
Chambersburg PA
CBHW051655250726

48653CB00007B/2674